Dr Patrick Wisedoc

Science of Dance Therapy:

Boost Your Energy & Mood

Science of Dance Therapy:
Boost Your Energy & Mood

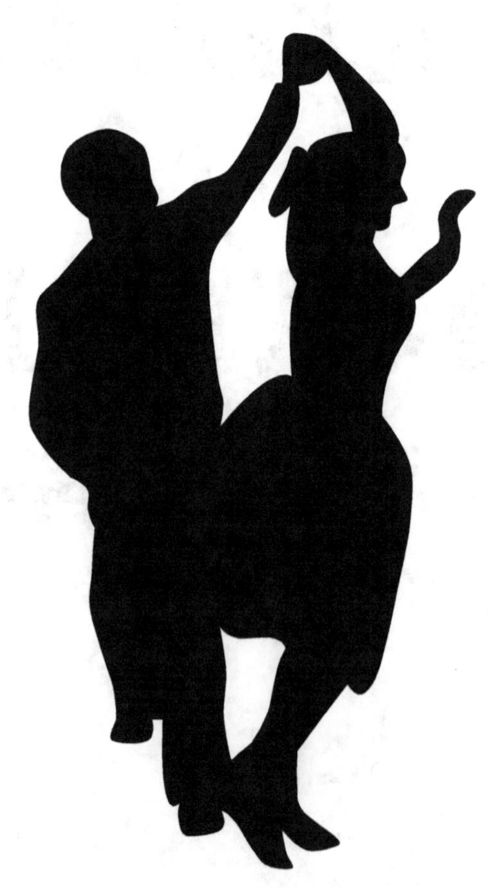

"Dance is the hidden language of the soul"

"You don't have to be great to dance, you just have to dance"

"In rhythm, there is healing"
"Dance with your troubles and they become your steps. "

"The body is a temple, movement is its prayer."

"Let your spirit take flight on the wings of rhythm."

"Every dancer tells a story, some with leaps, some with a sway."

"The soul that cannot speak can dance its truths."

"Find your rhythm, find yourself."

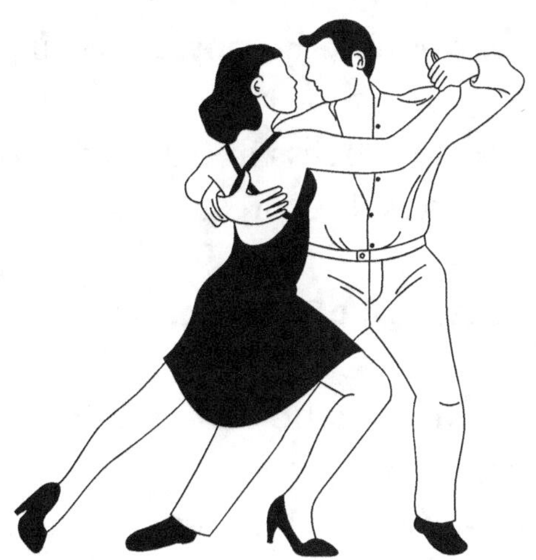

Contents

Contents

Chapter 4: The Body in Motion - Building Your Dance Foundation

Part 3: Music as Your Guide: Moving to the Beat

Chapter 5: The Power of Music for Health

Contents

Chapter 6: Dancing with the Music: Musicality in Dance

1. Rules for Dance (optional): Basic principles like posture and floor work
2. Breath: Connecting your breath to movement for flow and control
3. Design & Rhyme in Music: How music structure influences your dance

Part 4: Taking Your First Steps: Learning Dance the Healthy Way

Chapter 7: Movement Through Music: Starting Your Dance Journey

1. Beginning dance lesson: A step-by-step guide to get you started

Chapter 8: Exploring Dance Styles for You

1. A variety of dance styles presented, highlighting their benefits (consider including Cha Cha, Salsa, Polka, Tai Chi, as examples)

Contents

Introduction:

Imagine pirouetting with boundless energy, leaps fueled by unwavering strength, and a body that recovers swiftly. This isn't a fantasy; it's the reality within your grasp.

This book transcends the realm of typical dance guides. We delve into the fascinating world of dance science, specifically the intricate dance between your body's metabolism and peak performance.

Through the lens of cutting-edge research, we'll unveil the secrets to optimizing your fuel source – your diet. Forget restrictive fads and generic advice. We'll provide a personalized roadmap built on scientific evidence, empowering you to:

- Unleash Explosive Performance: Craft a customized fuel plan that unlocks your body's full potential, maximizing energy reserves and propelling your artistic expression.
- Sculpt Your Physique, Naturally: Manage weight in a healthy, sustainable way through strategic nutrition, ensuring a dancer's physique that's both aesthetically pleasing and functionally strong.
- Recover Like a Pro: Discover the power of targeted nutrients to accelerate recovery, minimize injuries, and keep you dancing day in and day out.
- Optimize Your Dance Metabolism: Gain a comprehensive understanding of the unique metabolic demands dancers face, allowing you to tailor your diet for unmatched results.

Introduction:

- Whether you're a seasoned professional gracing the stage or a passionate beginner embarking on your dance journey, this book equips you with the knowledge and tools to become the best dancer you can be. It's time to stop simply dancing – it's time to dance with science on your side.

Part 1: The Science Behind Dance Therapy
Chapter 1: Understanding Movement - The Science of
Kinesiology
1.1 Biomechanics: How your body moves (mechanics of joints, muscles, etc.)

Have you ever wondered how dancers achieve those seemingly impossible feats of grace and agility? The answer lies in the fascinating science of biomechanics, the study of how the body moves. It's the intricate interplay between your joints, muscles, and physics that allows you to leap, spin, and express yourself through movement.

The Building Blocks of Movement:

- **Joints**: These act as the connection points between your bones, allowing for a wide range of motion. Different joints, like the ball-and-socket joint in your shoulder or the hinge joint in your knee, offer varying degrees of flexibility and stability.

- **Muscles**: The powerhouses of movement! Muscles contract and relax, pulling on bones to create movement at the joints. Dancers rely heavily on different muscle groups depending on the style of dance.

- **Lever Systems**: The human body acts like a series of levers, with bones acting as levers and muscles applying the force. Understanding these lever systems allows dancers to maximize efficiency and power in their movements.

1.1 Biomechanics: How your body moves (mechanics of joints, muscles, etc.)

How Dance Utilizes Biomechanics:

- **Balance and Alignment:** Proper posture and alignment are crucial for efficient movement, injury prevention, and maximizing artistic expression. Biomechanics helps dancers understand ideal body positioning for different dance styles.

- **Range of Motion (ROM):** Dancers strive for a wide range of motion in their joints, allowing for impressive extensions, flexibility, and intricate footwork. Biomechanics principles help dancers train safely and effectively to improve their ROM.

- **Force Production and Control:** Powerful jumps and controlled landings require dancers to generate and control significant forces. Biomechanics helps dancers understand how to use their bodies to produce the necessary force with optimal technique.

- **Center of Gravity:** Maintaining a stable center of gravity is essential for balance and control. Biomechanics helps dancers understand how to shift their center of gravity for different dance movements.

1.1 Biomechanics: How your body moves (mechanics of joints, muscles, etc.)

Optimizing Your Dance Journey:

Understanding biomechanics empowers dancers to:

- **Reduce Injury Risk:** Proper technique based on biomechanics principles helps minimize stress on joints and muscles, preventing injuries.
- **Enhance Performance:** Knowing how your body moves allows for more efficient and powerful movements, leading to improved performance.
- **Maximize Training:** Biomechanics knowledge informs targeted exercises to strengthen specific muscle groups and improve weaknesses.
- **Biomechanics is more than just science;** it's the foundation for a safe, fulfilling, and expressive dance journey. By understanding how your body moves, you can unlock its full potential and take your dancing to new heights.

1.2 Anatomy: The building blocks of your movement (muscles, bones, etc.)

- **Focus on Muscle Groups:** Instead of just listing muscles and bones, mention specific muscle groups crucial for dance, like hamstrings for flexibility, glutes for power, and core muscles for stability.
- **Body Systems:** Briefly touch upon how other body systems like the nervous system (sends signals to muscles) and the respiratory system (delivers oxygen for movement) work together with bones and muscles for coordinated movement.
- **Movement Examples:** Connect anatomy to specific dance movements. For example, explain how strong core muscles help with balance in turns or how flexible hamstrings allow for deeper lunges.

Here's an example of how you could rewrite the sentence:

Anatomy: The Building Blocks of Your Movement

Just like a building needs a strong foundation, your body relies on its anatomical structure for movement. Muscles, the engines of movement, work in conjunction with bones, the framework of your body. Understanding key muscle groups like hamstrings, glutes, and core muscles will help you improve your dance technique and prevent injuries. Additionally, your nervous system sends signals to your muscles to coordinate movement, while your respiratory system delivers oxygen to keep your muscles fueled. By understanding how these systems work together, you can enhance your dance experience and appreciate the incredible mechanics of your body.

1.2 Anatomy: The building blocks of your movement (muscles, bones, etc.)

Anatomy: The Blueprint for Movement

Anatomy is the foundation of dance. It's the intricate blueprint that allows you to move with power, grace, and control. Understanding your body's structure, especially your muscles and bones, is crucial for maximizing your potential in dance therapy and minimizing the risk of injury.

Muscles: The Engines of Movement

Muscles are the powerhouses that drive your movement. Different muscle groups play specific roles in dance:

- **Core Muscles:** These muscles, including your abdominals, obliques, and lower back muscles, provide stability and support for your entire body. A strong core helps you maintain proper posture during dance and allows for more controlled movements.
- **Leg Muscles:** Powerful leg muscles like quadriceps (on the front of your thigh) and hamstrings (on the back) are crucial for jumping, leaps, and powerful kicks. Flexibility in these muscles is also vital for achieving a wider range of motion.
- **Foot and Ankle Muscles:** Strong foot and ankle muscles provide stability and balance, especially when performing intricate footwork or standing on pointe (ballet shoes with a strengthened shank).

1.2 Anatomy: The building blocks of your movement (muscles, bones, etc.)

- **Upper Body Muscles:** Don't forget your upper body! Muscles like shoulders, chest, and back contribute to posture, arm movements, and overall coordination.

By understanding the function of these key muscle groups, you can target specific areas for strengthening and stretching in your dance therapy program. This targeted approach will help you improve your technique, enhance your dance expression, and reduce the risk of muscle strain or imbalances.

Bones: The Framework for Movement

Bones provide the rigid framework that supports your body and allows for movement at your joints. In dance, the focus is often on the major joints like hips, knees, ankles, and shoulders. The flexibility and strength of these joints are crucial for performing dance movements safely and effectively.

For example, understanding the structure of your hip joint helps you achieve proper turnout (external rotation of the leg from the hip). Similarly, understanding the knee joint allows you to safely execute jumps and landings.

1.2 Anatomy: The building blocks of your movement (muscles, bones, etc.)

Nervous System: The Conductor of Movement

While muscles provide the power, your nervous system acts as the conductor. It sends signals from your brain to your muscles, coordinating movement and allowing for precise control. When you practice dance movements repeatedly, you create neural pathways in your brain, improving your coordination and making the movements feel more natural. This is why dance therapy can be so effective in improving motor skills and overall well-being.

Synergy: It's All Connected

Anatomy isn't just about individual muscles and bones. It's about how these systems work together. In dance, strong core muscles provide a stable base for powerful leg movements. Flexible hamstrings allow for deeper lunges, and a strong upper body contributes to balanced jumps. Understanding this interconnectedness is key to mastering dance movements and experiencing the joy of moving your body with intention.

1.3 Physiology: How your body functions during movement (cardiovascular, respiratory systems)

Physiology: The Engine Room of Movement

While anatomy provides the structure for movement, physiology delves into how your body's internal systems function to keep you moving. Dance therapy, with its focus on increased movement, puts a specific demand on two key physiological systems: the cardiovascular system and the respiratory system.

The Cardiovascular System: Your Internal Pump

Imagine your cardiovascular system as an intricate pump. The heart, the powerful muscle at its center, acts as the pump, circulating blood throughout your body. Blood carries oxygen and nutrients to your muscles, which are essential for movement. During dance therapy, your heart rate increases to deliver more oxygenated blood to your working muscles. This increased blood flow also helps remove waste products like carbon dioxide, keeping your muscles functioning optimally.

When you engage in dance therapy, you'll likely experience a noticeable increase in your heart rate. This is a normal response, and as your fitness level improves, your body becomes more efficient at delivering oxygen to your muscles, allowing you to sustain higher levels of activity for longer durations.

1.3 Physiology: How your body functions during movement (cardiovascular, respiratory systems)

- **The Respiratory System:** Delivering the Fuel

Your respiratory system, often referred to as your breathing system, works hand-in-hand with your cardiovascular system. It's responsible for taking in oxygen from the air and releasing carbon dioxide, a waste product from cellular respiration (the process by which your body converts food into energy).

During dance therapy, your breathing rate increases to meet the increased oxygen demands of your working muscles. You'll likely find yourself taking deeper breaths to ensure your body has enough oxygen to sustain your movements. Dance therapy can also help improve your lung capacity over time, allowing you to take in more oxygen with each breath, further enhancing your performance.

The Synergy Between Systems

The beauty of the human body lies in how different systems work together. During dance therapy, your cardiovascular system delivers oxygen-rich blood to your muscles, fueled by the oxygen your respiratory system takes in. This coordinated effort allows you to move with power, grace, and endurance.

Understanding these physiological processes can help you appreciate the incredible adaptability of your body and the positive impact dance therapy can have on your overall health. It can improve your cardiovascular health, increase your lung capacity, and boost your overall fitness level.

1.4 Exercise Physiology: The science of exercise and its impact on the body

Exercise physiology is the science that explores how the body adapts and responds to physical activity. This knowledge is crucial for understanding how dance therapy impacts your body and mind. Here's how dance therapy leverages exercise physiology principles:

- **Improved Cardiovascular Health:** As explained earlier, dance therapy elevates your heart rate, mimicking the effects of cardio exercise. This strengthens your heart muscle, improves blood flow, and increases your lung capacity, all contributing to better cardiovascular health.
- **Enhanced Muscular Strength and Endurance**: Dance therapy involves repetitive movements that engage various muscle groups. Over time, these movements lead to increased muscle strength and endurance. This allows you to perform more complex dance routines and improve your overall fitness level.
- **Increased Bone Density:** Dance, particularly activities with high-impact landings (e.g., jumps), can stimulate bone growth and increase bone density. This is especially beneficial for preventing osteoporosis later in life.
- **Weight Management:** Dance therapy can be a fun and effective way to burn calories and manage weight. The combination of cardio and strength elements often found in dance routines leads to increased calorie expenditure.

1.4 Exercise Physiology: The science of exercise and its impact on the body

- **Improved Balance and Coordination:** Dance therapy requires precise coordination and balance to perform movements. Regular participation can significantly improve your balance and coordination, reducing the risk of falls and injuries in daily life.
- **Mental and Emotional Benefits**: Exercise physiology also explores the mind-body connection. Dance therapy stimulates the release of endorphins, the body's natural mood elevators, leading to reduced stress and anxiety. Additionally, the creative expression and sense of accomplishment from dance can positively impact self-esteem and overall well-being.

By understanding how exercise physiology principles apply to dance therapy, you can appreciate its multifaceted approach to improving your physical and mental health.

Neuroscience: The Symphony of Movement

Neuroscience, the study of the nervous system, sheds light on the fascinating ways your brain and body communicate during dance therapy. Movement is a complex interaction, and understanding the brain's role in this process reveals the incredible power of dance to impact your physical and mental well-being.

The Motor Cortex: Your Movement Maestro

The motor cortex, located in your brain, is the maestro that orchestrates your movements. It sends signals to your muscles, dictating which ones to engage and how much force to exert. When you learn a new dance move, your brain forms new neural pathways, essentially creating a map for your muscles to follow. With repetition in dance therapy, these pathways become stronger and more efficient, allowing you to perform movements with greater accuracy and fluidity.

The Sensory Cortex: Feeling the Music

The sensory cortex receives information from your body, including your muscles, joints, and skin. This feedback loop allows you to sense your body's position in space and adjust your movements accordingly. In dance therapy, this feedback becomes crucial for maintaining balance, coordinating movement with the music, and achieving a sense of flow.

The Mirror Neuron System: Moving in Harmony

The mirror neuron system is a fascinating group of brain cells that activate when you observe someone else perform an action. These neurons are believed to play a role in empathy and learning by imitation. In dance therapy, the mirror neuron system might be involved in mimicking the instructor's movements or synchronizing your movements with other participants, fostering a sense of connection and community.

The Dopamine Connection: The Reward of Movement

Dance therapy can be a joyful and energizing experience. Part of this positive feeling stems from the release of dopamine, a neurotransmitter associated with reward and motivation. As you learn new dance moves and experience success in dance therapy, your brain releases dopamine, reinforcing the positive experience and motivating you to continue.

1.5 Neuroscience: The brain-body connection in movement

A Symphony of Body and Mind

Neuroscience highlights the beautiful dance between your brain and body. Dance therapy activates various brain regions, promoting motor learning, sensory integration, and emotional well-being. By understanding this connection, you can appreciate how dance therapy goes beyond physical movement to impact your cognitive function, mood, and overall brain health.

2.1 Dance movement psychotherapy: Exploring emotions through dance

Dance Movement Psychotherapy: Unveiling Your Inner World Through Movement

Dance movement psychotherapy (DMT) is a powerful form of therapy that utilizes the language of movement to explore your emotions, improve your mental health, and enhance your well-being. Unlike traditional talk therapy, DMP doesn't rely solely on verbal communication. Instead, it uses movement as a tool for self-expression and exploration.

The Power of Movement to Express Emotions

Words can sometimes fail to capture the full spectrum of our emotions. Dance, on the other hand, provides a direct and uncensored way to express what might be difficult to articulate verbally. Here's how DMP utilizes movement for emotional exploration:

- **Body Language as a Window to the Soul:** Our bodies often hold onto unspoken emotions. In DMP, you'll explore your natural movements and how they relate to your emotional state. Tightness in your shoulders might indicate tension, while fluid, expansive movements could signify joy. By observing your body language, you can gain valuable insights into your emotions.

2.1 Dance movement psychotherapy: Exploring emotions through dance

- **Movement as a Release Valve:** Sometimes, strong emotions need an outlet. DMP provides a safe space to express anger, sadness, or frustration through movement. You might stomp your feet, jump with abandon, or shake your body vigorously. This physical release can help you process and move through difficult emotions.
- **Moving Through Emotions:** DMP doesn't just allow you to express emotions; it can also help you move through them. The therapist might guide you through specific movement exercises designed to explore a particular emotion and then transition to more positive or neutral movements. This process can help you release pent-up emotions and find a more balanced emotional state.

Beyond Expression: The Benefits of DMP

While emotional exploration is a key aspect of DMP, its benefits extend far beyond:

- **Improved Self-Awareness:** By exploring movement and its connection to your emotions, you gain a deeper understanding of yourself. You learn to recognize your emotional triggers and develop healthier coping mechanisms.
- **Enhanced Body-Mind Connection:** DMP strengthens the connection between your body and mind. You become more aware of how your body responds to emotions and how movement can influence your mental state.

2.1 Dance movement psychotherapy: Exploring emotions through dance

- **Stress Reduction:** The physical release and emotional processing facilitated by DMP can significantly reduce stress and anxiety.
- **Greater Confidence:** As you gain comfort expressing yourself through movement and overcome emotional challenges, your confidence and self-esteem can blossom.
- **Social Connection:** DMP can be practiced in group settings, fostering a sense of connection and community with others who are also on their therapeutic journey.

Dance Movement Psychotherapy: A Journey of Self-Discovery

DMP isn't about achieving perfect dance skills; it's about using movement as a tool for self-discovery and emotional healing. Whether you're a seasoned dancer or have no prior experience, DMP welcomes you to explore your inner world through movement and experience the profound impact it can have on your emotional well-being.

2.2 **The creative-artistic process in dance/movement therapy: Using movement for self-expression and healing**

Dance/movement therapy (DMT) isn't just about prescribed exercises; it's a creative journey of self-discovery and healing through movement. This chapter delves into the core of DMT – the creative-artistic process. We'll explore how movement becomes a tool for self-expression, allowing you to tap into your inner creativity and unlock its potential for healing.

Beyond Technique: Unlocking Creativity in Movement

Unlike traditional dance classes focused on technical perfection, DMT prioritizes self-expression. Here's how the creative process unfolds:

- **Free Exploration:** The therapist might begin by creating a safe and supportive space where you can freely explore movement without judgment. You might experiment with walking, jumping, swaying, or spontaneous movements that arise from within.
- **Movement as Storytelling:** As you explore movement, the therapist might encourage you to use it to tell a story, express an emotion, or depict a memory. This process allows you to bypass verbal limitations and tap into a deeper, more personal level of expression.
- **Imagery and Metaphor:** The therapist might guide you to use imagery and metaphors to connect your movement to your internal world. For instance, envisioning yourself as a strong tree during challenging moments or expressing joy through light, flowing movements.

2.2 The creative-artistic process in dance/movement therapy: Using movement for self-expression and healing

- **Collaboration and Improvisation:** DMT can be a collaborative experience. The therapist might join you in movement or create prompts to spark improvisation. This allows for a deeper connection with the therapist and fosters a sense of playfulness and discovery.

The Healing Power of Creative Expression

The creative-artistic process in DMT promotes healing in various ways:

- **Emotional Release:** By using movement to express emotions you might struggle to verbalize, DMT provides a cathartic release. Suppressed anger, sadness, or frustration can find an outlet through powerful movements, promoting emotional healing.
- **Increased Self-Awareness:** As you explore your creative movement vocabulary, you gain a deeper understanding of your emotional landscape and how your body responds to these emotions. This self-awareness empowers you to make healthier choices in response to your emotional triggers.
- **Problem-Solving Through Movement:** The creative process allows you to explore challenges and conflicts through movement metaphors. For example, depicting a struggle in your life through a dance routine might help you identify new ways to navigate the situation.

2.2 The creative-artistic process in dance/movement therapy: Using movement for self-expression and healing

- **Building Confidence:** The act of expressing yourself creatively and witnessing the beauty of your own movement fosters self-acceptance and confidence. This newfound confidence can spill over into other aspects of your life.

Embracing Your Inner Artist

DMT doesn't require prior dance experience. The creative process welcomes everyone, regardless of skill level. It's about embracing the joy of movement and using it as a powerful tool for self-discovery, expression, and ultimately, healing. By participating in DMT, you embark on a journey of creative exploration, allowing your inner artist to emerge and guide you towards greater emotional well-being and a deeper connection with yourself.

3.1 Therapeutic and kinesthetic dance: Different styles of dance used for therapy

Dance/Movement Therapy (DMT) isn't confined to a single style. Instead, it utilizes the diverse language of dance to cater to individual needs and preferences. This chapter delves into the world of therapeutic and kinesthetic dance, exploring various styles often used in DMT sessions:

The Beauty of Choice: Matching Styles to Needs

The beauty of DMT lies in its flexibility. Unlike a traditional dance class, where everyone learns the same routine, the therapist works with you to find a style that resonates with your personality, goals, and physical abilities. Here's how different dance styles can be utilized for therapeutic purposes:

- **Modern Dance:** This expressive form of dance focuses on emotional exploration and internal landscapes. It allows you to connect with your inner world and express emotions through powerful, dynamic movements. It can be particularly helpful for those seeking emotional release or a deeper connection to their body.
- **Ballet:** While ballet might seem intimidating at first, its focus on posture, alignment, and controlled movements can be therapeutic. It promotes core strength, flexibility, and body awareness, all of which contribute to a sense of balance and control in life.

3.1 Therapeutic and kinesthetic dance: Different styles of dance used for therapy

- **Folk Dance:** Folk dances are often joyful and celebratory, emphasizing community and cultural connection. Engaging in such dances in a DMT session can foster a sense of belonging, reduce social isolation, and uplift your mood.
- **Improvisation**: Free improvisation allows you to move spontaneously, without following specific steps or choreography. It encourages creativity, self-expression, and problem-solving skills. Improvisation can be particularly helpful for those struggling with rigidity or difficulty expressing themselves verbally.
- **Contact Improvisation:** This unique style involves physical contact and partnering with others. It fosters trust, communication, and awareness of your body in relation to others. It can be beneficial for those seeking to improve social skills, build trust, and explore boundaries.
- **Yoga Flow:** While not strictly considered a dance style, yoga flow incorporates fluid, rhythmic movements that can be therapeutic. It promotes flexibility, relaxation, and body awareness, making it beneficial for stress reduction and improving physical well-being.

3.1 Therapeutic and kinesthetic dance: Different styles of dance used for therapy

Beyond Styles: The Power of Kinesthetic Dance

The term "kinesthetic" refers to the sense of movement and body awareness. Kinesthetic dance incorporates various styles but emphasizes the connection between movement, sensation, and emotions. Here's how it plays a role in DMT:

- **Mindful Movement:** Kinesthetic dance focuses on slowing down and experiencing the sensations of movement within your body. This mindfulness practice allows you to connect with your body's internal signals and create a deeper awareness of your emotional state.

- **Movement Exploration:** The therapist might guide you through specific movement tasks designed to explore different body parts, their range of motion, and the emotions associated with specific movements. This exploration can help you regain control over your body awareness and release any tension.

- **Embodiment:** Through kinesthetic dance, you practice embodying certain emotions or states of being. For example, focusing on expansive movements might evoke feelings of joy or confidence, while grounded, deliberate movements might cultivate a sense of stability. This embodiment process can positively impact your emotional well-being.

3.2 Dance therapy: Motion and emotion - The connection between movement and emotional well-being

Have you ever felt a surge of joy while dancing freely? Or perhaps experienced a release of tension through powerful movements? Dance therapy delves into the profound connection between movement and emotional well-being. It utilizes the language of your body to express emotions, improve mental health, and unlock a deeper sense of self.

The Body Speaks: Unveiling Emotions Through Movement

Words can sometimes fall short of capturing the full spectrum of our emotions. Dance therapy offers an alternative. It allows you to bypass verbal limitations and express yourself through movement:

- **Body Language as a Mirror:** Our bodies hold onto unspoken emotions. Tightly clenched fists might indicate anger, while fluid, expansive movements could signify joy. In dance therapy, you'll explore your natural movement patterns and how they relate to your emotional state.
- **Moving Through Emotions:** Dance therapy isn't just about expressing emotions; it can also help you move through them. The therapist might guide you through specific movement exercises designed to explore a particular emotion, followed by exercises promoting more positive or neutral movements. This process can help you release pent-up emotions and find a more balanced emotional state.

3.2 Dance therapy: Motion and emotion - The connection between movement and emotional well-being

- **The Power of Embodiment:** Through movement, you can embody certain emotions or states of being. For example, focusing on powerful, expansive movements might evoke feelings of confidence, while grounded, deliberate movements might cultivate a sense of stability. This embodiment process can positively impact your emotional well-being.

The Science Behind the Connection: How Movement Impacts Your Mind

The link between movement and emotions isn't just anecdotal; it's backed by science:

- **The Neurochemical Dance:** Physical activity releases endorphins, neurotransmitters often called the body's natural mood elevators. Dance therapy, with its focus on movement, can elevate your mood, reduce anxiety, and promote feelings of well-being.
- **Brain Plasticity:** Dance therapy stimulates the brain, promoting the formation of new neural pathways. This can improve cognitive function, memory, and emotional regulation.
- **Stress Reduction:** The rhythmic and repetitive nature of certain dance styles can be meditative and calming. This helps to reduce stress hormones like cortisol, promoting a sense of relaxation and emotional balance.

3.2 Dance therapy: Motion and emotion - The connection between movement and emotional well-being

The Benefits of Dance Therapy

Dance therapy goes beyond emotional release; it offers a holistic approach to well-being:

- **Improved Self-Awareness:** By exploring movement and its connection to emotions, you gain a deeper understanding of yourself. You learn to recognize your emotional triggers and develop healthier coping mechanisms.
- **Enhanced Body-Mind Connection**: Dance therapy strengthens the connection between your body and mind. You become more aware of how your body responds to emotions and how movement can influence your mental state.
- **Greater Confidence**: As you gain comfort expressing yourself through movement and overcome emotional challenges, your confidence and self-esteem can blossom.
- **Social Connection:** Dance therapy can be practiced in group settings, fostering a sense of connection and community with others who are also on their therapeutic journey.

3.2 Dance therapy: Motion and emotion - The connection between movement and emotional well-being

Dance Therapy: A Journey for Everyone

Whether you're a seasoned dancer or have no prior experience, dance therapy welcomes you. It's about embracing the joy of movement and using it as a powerful tool for self-discovery, emotional healing, and a deeper connection with your authentic self. So, take a step forward, explore the language of your body, and discover the transformative power of dance therapy.

4.1 The starting position for movement: Proper posture and alignment

Just like a house needs a solid foundation, your body needs proper posture and alignment before you embark on your dance therapy journey. In this chapter, we'll explore the starting position for movement, focusing on posture and alignment, to ensure you move safely, comfortably, and with optimal efficiency.

Finding Your Center: The Importance of Posture

Posture is your body's baseline position while standing. Good posture isn't just about looking "tall"; it plays a crucial role in:

- **Injury Prevention:** Proper posture distributes weight evenly across your joints, minimizing stress and reducing the risk of injuries. This is especially important when learning new dance movements.
- **Movement Efficiency:** Good posture allows your muscles to work optimally, facilitating smooth and efficient movement.
- **Balance and Coordination:** Balanced posture forms the foundation for good balance and coordination, crucial for dance activities.
- **Breathing:** Proper posture allows your lungs to expand fully, facilitating deeper breaths and improved oxygen intake, which is important for sustained movement.

4.1 The starting position for movement: Proper posture and alignment

Building Your Foundation: Key Elements of Good Posture

Here's a breakdown of key elements for good posture in the starting position:

- **Head**: Your head should be balanced on your spine, with your chin slightly tucked in and your gaze forward. Avoid looking down or tilting your head to the side.
- **Spine**: Imagine a long, neutral spine. Don't slouch or arch your back excessively. Engage your core muscles to maintain a stable and upright spine.
- **Shoulders**: Keep your shoulders relaxed and down, away from your ears. Avoid hunching or rounding your shoulders forward.
- **Arms**: Let your arms hang naturally at your sides with a slight bend at the elbows.
- **Hips**: Maintain a neutral hip position, avoiding excessive tilting forward or backward.
- **Knees**: Keep your knees slightly bent, not locked straight. This allows for better shock absorption and greater stability.
- **Feet**: Stand with your feet hip-width apart, toes pointed slightly outward. This provides a strong and stable base for movement.

4.1 The starting position for movement: Proper posture and alignment

Alignment: Creating Optimal Movement Patterns

Alignment refers to the proper positioning of your body parts for specific movements. Good alignment ensures:

- **Smooth, Controlled Movement:** Proper alignment promotes smooth transitions between movements and minimizes unnecessary strain on your muscles.
- **Prevention of Injuries:** Maintaining proper alignment during dance movements helps protect your joints and muscles from injury.

Finding Your Alignment: Tips for Beginners

Here are some tips for aligning your body in the starting position:

- Imagine a Line of Energy: Visualize a line of energy running from the crown of your head down through your spine and out through your feet. This helps you maintain a long and balanced posture.
- Body Awareness Exercises: Practice gentle body awareness exercises to improve your kinesthetic sense (sense of body movement). This allows you to feel how your body is positioned in space.
- Mirror Work: Utilize mirrors to observe your posture and alignment from different angles. This can help you identify areas needing improvement.

**4.1 The starting position for movement: Proper
posture and alignment**

Listen to Your Body: Finding Balance Between Structure and Freedom

While good posture and alignment are crucial, dance therapy also encourages freedom of movement. The key is to find a balance between structure and freedom. Here's how:

- **Be Mindful and Gentle:** As you refine your posture and alignment, be gentle with yourself. It takes time and practice to develop muscle memory and achieve optimal alignment.
- **Don't Force It**: If you experience pain, stop and consult a qualified dance therapist or healthcare professional. Dance therapy should be a joyful experience, not a source of discomfort.

Ready to Move Forward

By focusing on proper posture and alignment in the starting position, you create a strong foundation for safe and efficient movement in dance therapy. As you develop your body awareness and practice different dance styles, your posture and alignment will naturally improve. Remember, the journey is just as important as the destination. Embrace the learning process, enjoy the joy of movement, and experience the transformative power of dance therapy!

4.2 The geometry of the human body: Understanding your body's limitations and strengths

The human body, with its intricate structure and diverse capabilities, can be viewed through the lens of geometry. Understanding this geometry helps us appreciate our body's strengths and limitations in dance therapy.

Building Blocks: The Skeletal System as Framework

Our bones, forming the skeletal system, provide the rigid framework for movement. The geometry of our joints, determined by how bones connect, dictates the range of motion available in different parts of the body. Here's how geometry plays a role:

- **Ball-and-Socket Joints:** These joints, like the shoulder joint, offer a wide range of motion in multiple planes (think of a ball moving within a socket). This allows for circular movements, arm abduction (raising your arm to the side), and adduction (bringing your arm back down).
- **Hinge Joints:** Hinge joints, like the knee joint, allow movement in one plane (think of a door hinge). They provide stability for activities like walking, jumping, and bending.
- **Gliding Joints:** These joints, like those in your spine and wrists, allow for small, sliding movements. They contribute to overall flexibility and spinal mobility.

4.2 The geometry of the human body: Understanding your body's limitations and strengths

Understanding these joint geometries helps you:

- Maximize Your Range of Motion: By understanding how your joints move, you can explore movements within their safe range, optimizing your flexibility and expressive potential in dance therapy.
- Respect Your Limits: Knowing the limitations of your joints helps you avoid overextension or movements that could cause injury.

Muscles: The Engines and Levers

Muscles, attached to bones at various points, act as the engines that generate movement. Here's how muscle geometry impacts dance:

- **Lever Systems:** Muscles act on bones like levers, creating force and movement. The length and orientation of muscle fibers influence the leverage and power generated by specific muscle groups. For example, the quadriceps on the front of your thigh act as a lever to extend your knee for jumping.
- **Muscle Synergy:** Dance movements rarely involve isolated muscle activation. Multiple muscle groups work together synergistically to create coordinated and powerful movements. Understanding this synergy allows you to develop efficient movement patterns in dance therapy.

4.2 The geometry of the human body: Understanding your body's limitations and strengths

Knowing your muscle geometry can help you:

- Target Specific Muscle Groups: By understanding how muscle fibers are oriented, you can target specific muscles for strengthening and improving your dance technique.
- Develop Balance and Coordination: Training various muscle groups to work together in a coordinated manner is crucial for achieving balance and fluidity in dance movements.

Center of Gravity and Body Alignment

Our center of gravity (COG) is the point where all our body weight is concentrated. Maintaining a low center of gravity, often achieved by engaging your core muscles, contributes to:

- **Stability:** A low center of gravity provides a stable base for balance, allowing you to perform movements with greater control and precision.
- **Balance**: Maintaining your COG over your base of support (your feet) is crucial for preventing falls, especially during dynamic movements in dance therapy.

4.2 The geometry of the human body: Understanding your body's limitations and strengths

Understanding your COG can help you:

Improve Balance and Posture: By focusing on engaging your core and maintaining a low COG, you can improve your balance and overall posture, allowing for safer and more confident movement.
Master Turns and Spins: Maintaining a low COG is crucial for executing smooth turns and spins in dance therapy.

Beyond Geometry: It's All Connected

The human body is more than just a collection of geometric shapes. It's a complex system where everything is interconnected. Strong core muscles provide stability for powerful leg movements, while flexibility in your hamstrings allows for deeper lunges.

By understanding the geometry of your body, you gain valuable insights into its strengths and limitations. This empowers you to approach dance therapy with greater awareness, allowing you to explore movement possibilities within your safe range and maximize your potential for growth and emotional expression.

4.2 The geometry of the human body: Understanding your body's limitations and strengths

Embrace the Journey: From Limitations to Creative Exploration

While some limitations might exist due to our skeletal and muscular structure, dance therapy isn't about achieving perfect form. It's about celebrating the unique geometry of your body and using movement as a tool for self-discovery and emotional expression. Focus on what your body can do, explore creative movement possibilities within your safe range, and allow the joy of movement to guide you on your dance therapy journey.

4.3 The nomenclature of movement: Learning the language of dance terminology

Dance therapy isn't just about moving your body; it's about using movement as a form of communication. Just like any language, dance has its own vocabulary – a system of terms used to describe specific movements. Understanding this movement terminology empowers you to:

- **Follow Instructions Clearly:** During dance therapy sessions, the therapist might guide you through specific movements using terminology. A grasp of these terms allows you to follow instructions accurately and participate fully in the session.
- **Expand Your Movement Repertoire**: Learning new dance terms introduces you to a wider range of movements, enriching your movement vocabulary and enhancing your expressive potential in dance therapy.
- **Communicate Effectively:** As you progress in dance therapy, you might even start using movement terminology to describe your own movement experiences and creations.

4.3 The nomenclature of movement: Learning the language of dance terminology

Breaking Down the Basics: Common Dance Terminology

Dance terminology can be vast, but here's a breakdown of some fundamental terms you might encounter in dance therapy:

- **Locomotion:** These terms describe movements that travel through space, such as walk, run, skip, jump, hop, leap, slide, and gallop.
- **Directional Terms:** These terms indicate the direction of movement, such as forward, backward, sideways, diagonal, up, and down.
- **Levels:** These terms describe the height of your body in relation to the floor, such as high (on pointe), medium (standing upright), and low (close to the floor).
- **Turns and Spins:** These terms describe rotational movements, such as pirouette (a full turn on one leg), turn (a full rotation on both legs), and sashay (a walking turn with a hip sway).
- **Jumps and Leaps:** These terms describe movements where you propel yourself into the air, such as jump (a straight vertical leap), leap (a jump with a horizontal travel distance), and grand jeté (a large leap with legs split in mid-air).

4.3 The nomenclature of movement: Learning the language of dance terminology

- **Arm Movements:** These terms describe movements of the arms, such as port de bras (carriage of the arms), plié (bending the knees while raising the arms overhead), and arabesque (standing on one leg with the other leg extended behind and arms outstretched).

Beyond the Basics: Exploring Different Styles

As you delve deeper into dance therapy, you might encounter terminology specific to different dance styles. Here are some examples:

- **Ballet:** Développé (unfolding the leg from the hip), dégagé (pointed foot brushing the floor), and assemblé (a jumping step with legs assemblée – brought together – in mid-air).
- **Modern Dance:** Contraction (pulling the navel towards the spine), release (letting go of muscular tension), and improvisation (creating spontaneous movement).
- **Jazz Dance:** Kick ball change (alternating kicking one leg forward while the other foot steps), grapevine (a side-stepping pattern), and shimmy (a shaking movement of the shoulders and torso)..

4.3 The nomenclature of movement: Learning the language of dance terminology

Finding Your Voice: Moving Beyond Terminology

While dance terminology is a valuable tool, dance therapy isn't about achieving technical perfection. It's about using movement as a form of personal expression. Don't be afraid to explore intuitive movements and create your own movement vocabulary to express your unique emotions and experiences.

Embrace the Journey: From Understanding to Self-Expression

Learning dance terminology is an ongoing process. As you participate in dance therapy sessions and explore different styles, you'll gradually expand your movement vocabulary. Embrace the journey of learning, and remember that the most important aspect of dance therapy is using movement to connect with yourself and express your inner world authentically.

4.4 Adapting movement and dance therapy: Modifications for different abilities

Dance therapy is a beautiful practice that celebrates the power of movement for emotional well-being. However, the beauty of dance therapy lies in its inclusivity. It's not a one-size-fits-all approach; it can be adapted to cater to various abilities and limitations. This chapter explores how dance therapy can be modified to ensure everyone has the opportunity to experience the joy and benefits of movement.

Understanding Needs: Assessing Individual Abilities

The first step in adapting dance therapy is to understand the individual's needs and abilities. A qualified dance therapist will conduct an assessment that considers factors such as:

- **Physical limitations:** This could include range of motion limitations, balance issues, or strength deficits.
- **Cognitive abilities:** Some participants might require clearer instructions or benefit from visual cues.
- **Sensory sensitivities:** Certain individuals might be sensitive to loud music or bright lights, requiring adjustments to the therapy environment.

4.4 Adapting movement and dance therapy: Modifications for different abilities

Creative Modifications: Making Dance Therapy Accessible

Here are some creative ways to adapt dance therapy for different abilities:

- **Seated Dance**: For individuals who cannot stand for extended periods, dance therapy can be adapted to incorporate seated movements using chairs or supportive props. Arm movements, torso twists, and footwork variations can all be explored while seated.
- **Props and Assistive Devices**: Props like scarves, balls, and canes can be used to enhance balance, support movement exploration, and add a playful element to the therapy session.
- **Modified Movements**: The therapist can modify traditional dance moves to make them accessible for individuals with specific limitations. For example, jumps can be replaced with stomps or steps, and large arm movements can be adapted into smaller, more controlled gestures.
- **Focus on Breath and Body** Awareness: Dance therapy isn't just about grand movements. Focusing on breathwork, body scans, and gentle stretches can be incredibly therapeutic and promote relaxation and self-awareness.

4.4 Adapting movement and dance therapy: Modifications for different abilities

- **Partner Work Adaptations:** Partner work, a common element in dance therapy, can be adapted for individuals with limited mobility. This could involve gentle mirroring exercises or hand-holding for support during balance challenges.

Benefits for Everyone: The Power of Inclusive Dance Therapy

Adapting dance therapy doesn't diminish its benefits. Here's how everyone can gain from this inclusive approach:

- **Improved Emotional Expression:** Regardless of ability, movement provides a powerful outlet for expressing emotions. Adapted dance therapy allows everyone to participate in this process and experience emotional release.
- **Enhanced Body Awareness:** The act of focusing on movement, even in modified forms, fosters greater body awareness and proprioception (sense of body position).
- **Social Connection and Community:** Dance therapy, even in its adapted forms, can be a social experience. Group sessions can foster a sense of community and belonging for participants with diverse abilities.
- **Building Confidence:** Overcoming challenges and experiencing the joy of movement through adapted dance therapy can boost self-confidence and empower individuals.

4.4 Adapting movement and dance therapy: Modifications for different abilities

The Beauty of Dance: A Celebration of Individuality

Dance therapy, through its adaptability, celebrates the unique potential of every individual. It embraces the language of movement, not as a measure of physical prowess, but as a tool for self-discovery, emotional expression, and connection. So, whether you can move with grand leaps or gentle sways, dance therapy offers a space for you to explore your inner world and experience the transformative power of movement.

5.1 Rhythm: The heartbeat of music and its impact on movement

In dance therapy, movement and music are intricately linked. Music provides the soundtrack for your emotional journey, while rhythm serves as the heartbeat that guides your movements. Understanding rhythm and its impact is crucial for getting the most out of your dance therapy experience.

Breaking Down Rhythm: The Language of Beats

Rhythm is the underlying organizational pattern of music, created by the regular recurrence of beats and accents. It's like the pulse that drives the music forward. Here's a breakdown of key rhythmic elements:

- **Tempo**: This refers to the speed of the music, measured in beats per minute (BPM). Upbeat tempos can evoke feelings of joy and energy, while slower tempos can create a sense of calm and introspection.
- **Beat**: The basic unit of musical time, often felt as a pulse or a steady tick. In dance therapy, movements can be synchronized with the beat or create interesting counter-rhythms.
- **Accent**: A stronger emphasis on a particular beat, creating a sense of variation and interest within the rhythm. Dance movements can accentuate these accents for dramatic effect.
- **Time Signature**: This indicates the number of beats per measure and the type of note that receives one beat. While not essential for basic participation, understanding time signatures can help dancers anticipate changes in rhythm and create more complex movement patterns.

5.1 Rhythm: The heartbeat of music and its impact on movement

Rhythm's Impact on Movement: Moving to the Music

Rhythm has a profound impact on how we move:

- **Entrainment:** Our bodies naturally tend to synchronize with the rhythm of the music. Faster tempos might lead to jumps and energetic movements, while slower tempos might evoke more flowing, sustained movements.
- **Emotional Connection:** Different rhythms can evoke specific emotions. A fast, driving rhythm might make you feel excited, while a slow, melancholic rhythm might evoke feelings of sadness or longing. Dance therapy utilizes this connection to help you explore and express your emotions through movement.
- **Movement Quality:** Rhythm can influence the quality of your movement. Upbeat tempos might inspire sharp, energetic movements, while slower tempos might encourage smoother, more sustained movements.

5.1 Rhythm: The heartbeat of music and its impact on movement

Exploring Rhythm in Dance Therapy

Here are some ways rhythm is explored in dance therapy:

- **Matching Movements to Beats:** The therapist might guide you to synchronize your movements with the beat of the music, clapping, stomping, or jumping on specific beats.
- **Creating Counter-rhythms:** You might experiment with moving against the beat, creating tension and release or a sense of playfulness.
- **Following Musical Accents:** The therapist might encourage you to accentuate your movements on specific beats, adding emphasis and exploring different movement dynamics.
- **Emotional Expression Through Rhythm:** Explore how different rhythms make you feel and use that connection to express your emotions through movement improvisation.

Finding Your Groove: The Importance of Personal Connection

While rhythm plays a crucial role in dance therapy, it's not about achieving perfect synchronization. It's about finding a personal connection to the music and allowing the rhythm to guide your movement in a way that feels authentic and emotionally expressive.

5.1 Rhythm: The heartbeat of music and its impact on movement

Embrace the journey of discovery, and don't be afraid to experiment with different rhythms and movement possibilities. The joy of movement and the power of emotional expression are at the heart of dance therapy, regardless of your dance expertise.

5.2 Melody: The emotional language of music

In dance therapy, music isn't just background noise; it's a powerful tool for emotional expression and movement exploration. While rhythm provides the structure and heartbeat, melody, the succession of musical notes, acts as the emotional language that guides your movement journey.

The Power of Melody: Evoking Emotions Through Sound

Melodies are like stories told through notes. They can evoke a wide range of emotions, from joy and excitement to sadness and longing. Here's how melody plays a role in dance therapy:

- **Emotional Connection:** Different melodies have the inherent ability to trigger specific emotions. A soaring melody might evoke feelings of hope and inspiration, while a minor key melody might create a sense of introspection and melancholy. The therapist might curate music with specific melodies to facilitate the exploration of particular emotions in the session.
- **Movement as Storytelling:** By responding to the emotional language of the melody with your movement, you can tell your own story. Energetic movements might reflect feelings of joy conveyed by the melody, while slower, more introspective movements might correspond to a melancholic melody.

5.2 Melody: The emotional language of music

- **Creating Movement Dynamics:** Melodies often have dynamic variations, with crescendos (building intensity) and decrescendos (softening intensity). Dance therapy can utilize these dynamics to create a flow of movement that mirrors the emotional journey of the melody. For example, jumping and expansive movements could correspond to crescendos, while flowing, grounded movements might reflect decrescendos.

Exploring Melody in Movement

Here are some ways to explore the emotional language of melody in dance therapy:

- **Movement Improvisation:** The therapist might play a piece of music with a distinct melody and encourage you to move freely in response to the emotions it evokes.
- **Mirroring the Melody:** Experiment with mirroring the rise and fall of the melody with your movements, using expansive gestures for high notes and more grounded movements for lower notes.
- **Movement Dialogue:** The therapist might play contrasting melodies and guide you to explore how your movement changes in response to the shift in emotional tone.

Beyond Technique: Finding Your Personal Expression

Dance therapy isn't about perfectly interpreting every musical nuance. It's about allowing the melody to resonate with you and using your movement to express the emotions it evokes. Here's why personal connection is key:

- **Subjective Experience:** The emotions triggered by a melody can be subjective. What evokes joy in one person might create a sense of nostalgia in another. Trust your own experience and move in a way that feels authentic to you.
- **Movement Vocabulary:** Don't be limited by technical dance skills. Your movement vocabulary can be as simple as walking, swaying, or reaching, as long as it allows you to express the emotions stirred by the melody.

The Symphony of Movement and Emotion

Melody and movement create a beautiful synergy in dance therapy. By allowing the melody to guide your emotions and using your body to express those emotions, you embark on a powerful journey of self-discovery and emotional release. Embrace the music, feel the emotions, and let your body move freely, creating your own unique dance narrative.

5.3 Harmony: Creating balance and depth in music

Music in dance therapy isn't just about melody and rhythm; it's a rich tapestry woven with multiple layers of sound. Harmony, the way different notes and chords interact to create a cohesive whole, plays a crucial role in shaping the emotional landscape of the music and your movement experience.

Understanding Harmony: The Chords that Color the Music

Harmony refers to the concurrent use of multiple pitches (notes) to create chords. These chords, and the way they progress throughout a piece of music, significantly impact the overall feel and mood. Here's a breakdown of key harmonic elements:

- **Chords**: A combination of notes played together, creating a specific sound. Chords can be consonant (pleasing and harmonious) or dissonant (creating tension and unease).
- **Chord Progressions:** The sequence in which chords change throughout the music. These progressions can evoke a sense of stability, resolution, tension, or release, depending on the chords chosen and their order.
- **Musical Texture:** This refers to the overall thickness or density of the music, influenced by the number of instruments playing and the complexity of the chords. A thicker texture with multiple instruments playing complex chords can create a sense of fullness and richness, while a thinner texture with simpler chords might feel more sparse and open.

5.3 Harmony: Creating balance and depth in music

Harmony's Impact on Movement:

Harmony, both through chords and overall texture, plays a role in dance therapy by:

- **Shaping Emotional Expression:** Different chords and progressions evoke distinct emotions. A major key progression might create feelings of joy and optimism, while a minor key progression might evoke sadness or introspection. The therapist might use music with specific harmonies to target particular emotions in a session.

- **Creating Movement Dynamics:** Similar to melody, harmonies can have dynamic variations. The therapist might guide you to explore movement that reflects these changes, using powerful movements for dissonant chords and more flowing movements for resolved chords.

- **Adding Depth and Complexity:** Harmony adds depth and complexity to the music, enriching your movement experience. You can explore a wider range of movement qualities, responding not just to the melody and rhythm but also to the subtle nuances of the chords.

5.3 Harmony: Creating balance and depth in music

Exploring Harmony in Movement

Here are some ways to explore the role of harmony in dance therapy:

- Movement Improvisation with Chord Changes: The therapist might play music with distinct chord progressions and guide you to improvise movements that shift in response to the changing harmonies. For example, tense, angular movements for dissonant chords and expansive, flowing movements for resolved chords.
- Focusing on Musical Texture: Explore how the density of the music (number of instruments playing) influences your movement choices. Dense textures might inspire more complex movements, while sparse textures might encourage simpler, more focused movements.
- Movement Dialogue with Harmony: The therapist might play contrasting sections of music with different harmonies and guide you to explore how your movement dialogue changes in response to the shift in the sonic landscape.

5.3 Harmony: Creating balance and depth in music

Beyond the Notes: Feeling the Emotional Journey

While understanding basic harmony can enhance your experience, dance therapy isn't about music theory analysis. It's about feeling the emotional journey of the music and using your movement to express those emotions:

- **Intuitive Response:** Trust your intuition and allow the harmonies to resonate with you on an emotional level. Move in a way that feels authentic and reflects the way the music makes you feel.
- **Movement Exploration:** Don't be afraid to experiment with different movement qualities in response to the harmonies. There's no right or wrong way to move; the key is to find movement that allows you to express yourself freely.

The Symphony of Movement and Music

Harmony, along with melody and rhythm, completes the beautiful symphony of music that guides your movement in dance therapy. By allowing the music to touch you emotionally and using your body to express those emotions, you create a holistic and transformative experience. So, move freely, feel the music in all its layers, and let your body tell the story your emotions want to express.

5.4 Beat: The driving force that gets us moving

dance therapy - it's the driving force that gets us moving. It's like the steady pulse of the music that pulls our bodies into action. Here's a deeper dive into why beat is so important:

- **The Body's Natural Response:** Our bodies have an inherent tendency to synchronize with a beat. It's almost primal - think about tapping your foot or nodding your head to music. This natural entrainment makes beat the foundation for movement exploration in dance therapy.
- **Energy and Emotion:** Different tempos (speeds) of beats evoke distinct energies and emotions. A fast, driving beat can infuse your movements with joy and excitement, while a slow, steady beat might create a sense of calm and introspection. The therapist can curate music with specific beats to target particular emotional exploration in a session.
- **Structure and Freedom:** Beat provides a sense of structure in dance therapy. It acts as a guiding force, helping you stay connected to the music while allowing for creative freedom within the rhythm. You can explore different movement styles and qualities all while staying anchored to the beat.
- **Building Confidence:** Following the beat and feeling yourself move in sync with the music can be incredibly empowering. It fosters a sense of accomplishment and builds confidence in your ability to move and express yourself creatively.

5.4 Beat: The driving force that gets us moving

Exploring Beat in Dance Therapy:

Here are some ways dance therapy sessions might utilize the power of beat:

- **Matching Movements:** The therapist might guide you to synchronize basic movements like walking, jumping, or clapping with the beat of the music. This helps you connect with the rhythm and establish a foundation for further exploration.
- **Accenting the Beat:** You might experiment with accenting specific beats within the music with stronger or more dynamic movements. This adds emphasis and creates a playful dialogue between your movement and the musical structure.
- **Creating Counter-rhythms:** While most of the time movements might complement the beat, you can also explore moving against the beat. This can create a sense of tension and release, or add a layer of complexity to your movement vocabulary.
- **Building Stamina and Coordination:** Following a steady beat throughout a piece of music can improve your stamina and coordination. This can be especially beneficial for individuals who want to enhance their overall physical well-being through dance therapy.

5.4 Beat: The driving force that gets us moving

Finding Your Groove:

Remember, in dance therapy, the focus isn't on achieving perfect robotic precision. It's about finding your own groove, a comfortable and expressive way to move in response to the beat:

- **Feel the Rhythm:** Don't just listen to the beat; feel it in your body. Allow it to guide your movements naturally and intuitively.
- **Explore Different Styles**: The beauty of beat is its versatility. You can explore different dance styles, from the energetic stomps of African dance to the flowing arm movements of contemporary dance, all anchored by the beat.
- **Focus on Enjoyment:** Above all, focus on enjoying the experience of moving to the beat. Let the rhythm guide you, express yourself freely, and celebrate the joy of movement.

So, the next time you hear a catchy beat, don't just stand still. Let your body move, feel the rhythm take over, and experience the joy and emotional release that comes with dancing to the beat!

5.5 Musicality: Developing your sense of musicality and expression through dance

In dance therapy, musicality isn't just about following the beat; it's about cultivating a deeper connection between music and movement, using both as tools for emotional expression. It's about developing your ability to listen not just with your ears, but with your whole body.

The Essence of Musicality:

Musicality in dance therapy involves:

- **Understanding the Elements of Music:** A basic grasp of musical elements like rhythm, melody, harmony, and dynamics can enhance your ability to respond to the music with your movement. This knowledge allows you to move beyond simply matching the beat and delve deeper into the emotional landscape of the music.
- **Body Awareness and Kinesthetic Intelligence:** Being attuned to your body's sensations and how it moves in space is crucial for translating musical nuances into movement. The more aware you are of your body's potential, the richer and more expressive your movement vocabulary becomes.
- **Emotional Connection:** The ultimate goal of musicality in dance therapy is to connect with the emotions evoked by the music and express those emotions through your movement. Allow the music to resonate with you, and let your body move freely to tell your story.

5.5 Musicality: Developing your sense of musicality and expression through dance

Developing Your Musicality:

Here are some ways to cultivate your musicality in dance therapy:

- **Movement Improvisation:** Engage in frequent movement improvisation exercises where you respond freely to the music with your body. Don't be afraid to experiment and explore different movement qualities based on the emotions you feel from the music.
- **Body Mapping:** This technique involves focusing on specific body parts and exploring how they can move in response to different musical elements. For example, explore how your shoulders might react to a crescendo (building intensity) in the music.
- **Mirroring the Music:** Experiment with mirroring the rise and fall of the melody with your movements, or using expansive gestures for dynamic crescendos and more contracted movements for decrescendos.
- **Movement Dialogue:** The therapist might play contrasting pieces of music and guide you to explore how your movement dialogue changes with the shift in tempo, mood, and musical style.

5.5 Musicality: Developing your sense of musicality and expression through dance

Beyond Technique: The Power of Authenticity

While developing technical skills can enhance your musicality, it's not about achieving technical perfection. Here's why authenticity is key:

- Your Unique Voice: Everyone experiences music differently. Your movement expression should be authentic to your own emotions and how the music resonates with you. Don't try to copy someone else's style; find your own unique movement voice.
- Emotional Release: The power of musicality lies in using movement to express emotions that might be difficult to articulate with words. Allow yourself to be vulnerable and move freely without judgment.
- The Joy of Movement: Don't get bogged down in overthinking the music. Embrace the joy of moving your body and the freedom to express yourself through dance.

The Symphony of Self-Discovery

Musicality in dance therapy is a beautiful journey of self-discovery. By deepening your connection between music and movement, you unlock a powerful tool for emotional exploration and expression. Let the music guide you, embrace your unique movement voice, and celebrate the joy of moving your body to the soundtrack of your soul.

6.1 Rules for Dance : Basic principles like posture and floor work

While dance therapy prioritizes personal expression and emotional release over rigid rules, there are some basic principles that can enhance your experience and safety:

Posture:

- **Alignment:** Strive for a neutral spine with your shoulders relaxed and stacked over your hips. This promotes proper weight distribution and reduces strain on your back and joints.
- **Engagement:** Engage your core muscles to maintain good posture. This provides stability and support for your movements.
- **Elongation:** Imagine lengthening your spine upwards, creating a sense of space and openness in your body.

Floor Work:

- **Warm-up:** Always warm up your body before floor work to prepare your muscles and joints.
- **Support:** Utilize your arms and legs for support while on the floor. Don't put undue stress on your neck or back.
- **Body Awareness:** Be mindful of your body's limitations. Don't force yourself into uncomfortable positions that could lead to injury.
- **Exploration:** Explore different ways to move on the floor, such as rolling, crawling, lunging, and kneeling.

6.1 Rules for Dance : Basic principles like posture and floor work

Additional Considerations:

- Alignment with Breath: Coordinate your movements with your breath. Inhale as you open up and exhale as you contract or release.
- Safety: Listen to your body. If you experience any pain, stop the movement and consult your therapist.
- Respect for Space: Be mindful of your personal space and the space of others in a group setting.

Remember: These principles are guidelines, not rigid rules. The most important aspect of dance therapy is to move in a way that feels comfortable and authentic for you. Don't be afraid to experiment and explore different ways of moving within your safe range.

Here are some additional points to consider:

- Dance Therapy vs. Formal Dance Styles: Dance therapy doesn't require mastery of specific dance styles. It's about using movement for self-expression, not about achieving technical perfection.
- Focus on Feeling: While posture and floor work can enhance your experience, the primary focus should be on how the movement makes you feel and how it helps you express yourself.
- The Therapist's Role: A qualified dance therapist will guide you through these principles in a safe and supportive environment, tailoring them to your individual needs and abilities.

6.2 Breath: Connecting your breath to movement for flow and control

In dance therapy, breath is more than just air; it's the bridge between your mind and body, creating a flow of movement and a sense of control. Here's how breath work can elevate your dance therapy experience:

The Power of Breath:

- Connection: Breath connects your conscious mind with your physical body. By focusing on your breath, you become more aware of your movements and can control them with greater intention.
- Flow and Stamina: Coordinating your breath with movement creates a sense of flow and rhythm. Inhaling as you initiate movement and exhaling as you release provides sustained energy for longer dance sessions.
- Emotional Release: Breath can be a powerful tool for emotional release. Deep, controlled breaths can help you calm your nervous system and access deeper emotions that might be expressed through movement.

6.2 Breath: Connecting your breath to movement for flow and control

Breath and Movement Techniques:

Here are some techniques to explore the connection between breath and movement in dance therapy:

- Simple Breath Coordination: Start by synchronizing basic movements like walking or arm circles with your breath. Inhale as you initiate the movement and exhale as you complete it.
- Deep Breathing Exercises: Practice deep, diaphragmatic breaths where your belly expands with each inhale and contracts with each exhale. This can promote relaxation and focus.
- Breath Control for Movement Dynamics: Experiment with using breath to control the intensity of your movements. Inhale for expansive movements and exhale for contractions or releases.
- Emotional Expression through Breath: The therapist might guide you to explore how different emotions affect your breath. You can then use breath control to express those emotions through movement. For example, shallow, rapid breaths might represent anxiety, while slow, deep breaths might represent calmness.

6.2 Breath: Connecting your breath to movement for flow and control

Beyond Technique: Finding Your Breath

While there are techniques to explore, the key is to find a natural breath pattern that complements your movement:

- Listen to Your Body: Pay attention to your body's natural breathing rhythm and don't force a specific pattern. The breath should guide your movement, not the other way around.
- Focus on Feeling: Notice how your breath feels as you move. Does it become shallow when you feel stressed? Does it deepen when you feel relaxed? This awareness can help you use breath to regulate your emotions.
- No Right or Wrong: There's no single "correct" way to breathe in dance therapy. The most important thing is to find a breathing pattern that feels comfortable and allows you to move freely and express yourself authentically.

The Symphony of Movement and Breath

Breathwork adds another layer of depth and intentionality to your movement in dance therapy. By connecting your breath with your movement, you create a beautiful synergy between mind and body, promoting flow, control, and emotional expression. So, breathe deeply, feel the connection, and let your body move freely to the rhythm of your breath.

6.3 Design & Rhyme in Music: How music structure influences your dance

Music in dance therapy isn't just a random collection of sounds; it has a structure, a design, that can significantly influence your movement choices and emotional experience. Here's how understanding the building blocks of music can elevate your dance therapy journey:

Musical Design: The Blueprint for Movement

Music structure refers to the organized arrangement of musical elements like melody, rhythm, harmony, and form. Just like a building has a blueprint, music has an underlying structure that guides the listener's experience. Here are some key components of musical design that influence dance:

- **Phrases and Sections:** Music is often divided into smaller units called phrases, which are then grouped into larger sections. These phrases and sections create a sense of call and response, which can translate into your movement vocabulary. For example, a repeated musical phrase might inspire you to create a repetitive movement pattern.
- **Dynamics:** The intensity level of the music, indicated by markings like piano (soft) and forte (loud), can influence the energy and power of your movements. Loud crescendos (building intensity) might inspire jumps and expansive movements, while soft decrescendos (softening intensity) might encourage slower, controlled movements.

6.3 Design & Rhyme in Music: How music structure influences your dance

- **Form:** The overall structure of a piece of music, often represented by letters like AABA or ABAB, creates a sense of familiarity and anticipation. Recognizing these forms can help you structure your own movement improvisation within the framework of the music.

Rhyme in Music: Creating Predictability and Surprise

Musical rhyme refers to the repetition of musical ideas, like melodies or rhythmic patterns, throughout a piece. This repetition creates a sense of predictability and comfort, while variations on those ideas can introduce surprise and keep the listener engaged.

Here's how rhyme in music influences dance:

- **Movement Repetition:** Repeated musical phrases can inspire you to create repetitive movement patterns, establishing a foundation for your improvisation. You can then layer variations on those repetitive movements as the music introduces new elements.
- **Movement Anticipation:** By recognizing recurring musical themes, you can anticipate upcoming changes and structure your movement accordingly. For example, if you know a loud crescendo is coming, you might prepare for a jump or a powerful movement expression.

6.3 Design & Rhyme in Music: How music structure influences your dance

- **Movement Exploration:** Musical variations within a recurring theme offer opportunities for creative movement exploration. You can utilize these variations to add dynamics, introduce new movement qualities, or shift the emotional tone of your dance.

Beyond Structure: Finding Your Flow

Understanding musical structure and rhyme can enhance your dance therapy experience, but it shouldn't restrict your movement exploration:

- Intuitive Response: Don't get bogged down in over-analyzing every musical detail. Trust your intuition and allow the music to move you emotionally. Let your body respond naturally to the structure and flow of the music.
- Movement Freedom: While structure provides a framework, there's always space for improvisation and creative expression. Don't be afraid to break away from the expected and explore your own unique movement vocabulary.
- Focus on the Journey: The most important aspect is the experience of moving your body and expressing yourself freely. Enjoy the process of discovery as you explore the music and its influence on your movement.

6.3 Design & Rhyme in Music: How music structure influences your dance

The Symphony of Movement and Music

By understanding the design and rhyme within music, you gain a deeper appreciation for its structure and how it can influence your movement choices. This knowledge allows you to create a more dynamic and expressive dance experience in your dance therapy sessions. So, listen closely, feel the rhythm and structure, and let the music guide you on a beautiful journey of movement and emotional release.

7.1 Beginning dance lesson: A step-by-step guide to get you started

Welcome to the exciting world of dance! Whether you crave the grace of ballet or the energy of hip-hop, this guide will help you take your first steps.

Step 1: Ignite Your Passion

Explore Dance Styles: Salsa, hip-hop, ballet, tap, there are so many options! Watch videos or attend live performances to discover what resonates with you. Think about the music you enjoy and the kind of movement that excites you.

Step 2: Choose Your Path

- Class Time: Enrolling in a beginner's dance class provides a structured learning environment with a supportive instructor. Studios often offer trial classes, so you can test the waters before committing.
- Go Solo: If you prefer to learn at home, numerous online resources cater to beginners. Search for "[YouTube] beginner dance tutorials" in your chosen style.

Step 3: Prepare for Takeoff

- Dress for Success: Wear comfortable clothing that allows for free movement. Think loose-fitting clothes and supportive shoes.
- Embrace the Beat: Most dance styles are heavily influenced by music. Familiarize yourself with the rhythm and feel of the music you'll be dancing to.

7.1 Beginning dance lesson: A step-by-step guide to get you started

Step 4: Your First Lesson

- Warm Up: Just like any physical activity, a proper warm-up is crucial. Follow your instructor's lead or find some light stretches online.
- Master the Basics: Most styles begin with fundamental techniques like posture, footwork, and coordination. Focus on these building blocks for a strong foundation.
- Don't Be Shy: Everyone starts somewhere! Embrace mistakes as part of the learning process.
- Have Fun! Dance is about expressing yourself and enjoying the movement. Let loose, smile, and celebrate your progress.

Bonus Tip: Practice regularly, even if it's just for a few minutes each day. Repetition is key to building muscle memory and improving your skills.

Remember, the most important thing is to have fun and enjoy the journey. With dedication and a little practice, you'll be moving and grooving in no time!

A variety of dance styles presented, highlighting their benefits (consider including Cha Cha, Salsa, Polka, Tai Chi, as examples)

The world of dance offers a wealth of styles, each with unique benefits that go beyond just fancy footwork. Here's a taste of a few popular options to get your feet tapping:

- **Salsa:** This vibrant Latin dance is known for its sensual hip movements and lively footwork. Salsa is a fantastic way to improve cardiovascular health, burn calories, and boost coordination. Plus, the emphasis on partner connection can be a great way to meet new people and have a blast!

- **Cha Cha:** Cha Cha is another Latin dance that's perfect for beginners. The rhythmic, side-step movements are great for strengthening core muscles and improving balance. It's also a low-impact activity, making it accessible to people of all ages and fitness levels.

- **Polka:** This lively folk dance from Central Europe is known for its fast spins and joyful energy. The polka is a fantastic way to boost your mood, improve agility, and get your heart rate up. The simple steps and repetitive patterns make it easy for beginners to pick up.

- **Tai Chi:** While not typically considered a social dance, Tai Chi offers a unique blend of movement and meditation. The slow, graceful motions improve flexibility, balance, and posture. Tai Chi is also a great way to reduce stress, improve focus, and promote overall well-being.

A variety of dance styles presented, highlighting their benefits (consider including Cha Cha, Salsa, Polka, Tai Chi, as examples)

- This is just a small sampling! There are countless dance styles out there, each offering its own set of physical and mental benefits. So lace up your shoes, crank up the music, and discover the joy of movement!

Here are some additional styles to consider:

- **Ballet:** Builds strength, flexibility, and poise.
- **Hip-Hop:** Improves coordination, rhythm, and confidence.
- **Tap Dance:** Enhances musicality, footwork, and agility.

No matter your age, fitness level, or interests, there's a dance style out there waiting for you. So why not step out of your comfort zone and start grooving?

9.1 Diet for dancers: Nutritional needs for optimal performance

Dancers fuel their amazing feats with a carefully balanced diet. Here's a breakdown of their key nutritional needs for optimal performance:

- **Macronutrients**: These are the building blocks of energy.

- **Carbohydrates (55-60% of diet):** They provide the primary fuel source for muscles and the brain. Focus on complex carbs found in whole grains (brown rice, quinoa, oats), fruits, and vegetables. These offer sustained energy release compared to simple carbs like sugary drinks or white bread.

- **Protein** (15-20% of diet): Essential for muscle repair, growth, and recovery. Lean protein sources like chicken, fish, beans, lentils, tofu, and low-fat dairy are all excellent choices.

- **Healthy Fats** (20-30% of diet): Don't avoid fats! They provide energy, support hormone balance, and aid in vitamin absorption. Choose healthy fats from sources like nuts, seeds, avocados, and olive oil.

- **Micronutrients** (Vitamins *&* Minerals): These power various bodily functions.

9.1 Diet for dancers: Nutritional needs for optimal performance

- **Calcium and Vitamin D**: Crucial for strong bones to prevent stress fractures. Dairy products, leafy greens, fortified plant-based milk, and fatty fish are good sources.

- **Iron**: Carries oxygen to muscles, preventing fatigue. Lean red meat, poultry, fish, beans, lentils, and dark leafy greens are all iron-rich options.

- **B Vitamins**: Support energy metabolism and nervous system function. Whole grains, fruits, vegetables, and lean protein sources are packed with B vitamins.

Hydration:

Dancers lose a lot of fluids through sweat. Staying adequately hydrated is crucial for optimal performance and recovery. Aim to drink plenty of water throughout the day, even before feeling thirsty.

Sample Daily Meal Plan:

- **Breakfast**: Oatmeal with berries and nuts, Greek yogurt with granola and fruit

- **Lunch**: Grilled chicken breast on brown rice with roasted vegetables

- **Dinner**: Salmon with quinoa and steamed broccoli

9.1 Diet for dancers: Nutritional needs for optimal performance

- **Snacks**: Fruits with nut butter, vegetable sticks with hummus, yogurt with granola

Remember:

- This is a general guideline. Individual needs may vary depending on age, activity level, and dance style.
- Consult a registered dietitian or sports nutritionist for a personalized plan tailored to your specific needs.
- Listen to your body: Eat intuitively and adjust your portions based on your hunger cues and activity level.
- Fuel for performance: Eat a balanced meal 2-4 hours before practice or rehearsal.
- Refuel after workouts: Have a recovery snack within 30-60 minutes after dancing to replenish glycogen stores and aid muscle repair.

By following these tips and prioritizing a balanced diet, dancers can fuel their bodies for peak performance, improve recovery, and stay injury-free.

9.2 Caloric and nutrient intake: Understanding calorie needs and balancing nutrients

Dancers have unique energy demands. Unlike the average person, they require a specific balance of calories and nutrients to perform at their best, recover effectively, and avoid injuries.

Calorie Needs:

- **Estimating Your Base:** There's no one-size-fits-all answer, but a general starting point is 45-50 calories per kilogram of body weight for females and 50-55 calories per kilogram for males. This helps estimate the baseline calories needed for basic bodily functions.

- **Factor in Activity:** On top of the base, dancers need to consider their activity level. More intense training schedules or styles like ballet or hip-hop require additional calories to fuel the increased exertion.

Balancing Nutrients:

Once you have a ballpark calorie range, it's crucial to focus on the quality of those calories. Here's where macronutrients come in:

- Carbohydrates (55-60%): Your primary energy source. Prioritize complex carbs like whole grains, fruits, and vegetables for sustained energy.

9.2 Caloric and nutrient intake: Understanding calorie needs and balancing nutrients

- Protein (15-20%): Essential for muscle repair and growth. Lean protein sources like chicken, fish, beans, and low-fat dairy are key.

- Healthy Fats (20-30%): Don't skimp here! Fats provide energy, support hormone balance, and aid vitamin absorption. Choose healthy fats from nuts, seeds, avocados, and olive oil.

Micronutrients Matter:

While calories and macronutrients are essential, don't forget micronutrients (vitamins & minerals)! They power various functions and are crucial for dancers:

- Calcium & Vitamin D: Strong bones for injury prevention. Dairy, leafy greens, fortified plant-based milk, and fatty fish are good sources.

- Iron: Combats fatigue by carrying oxygen to muscles. Lean meats, poultry, fish, beans, lentils, and dark leafy greens are iron-rich.

- B Vitamins: Support energy metabolism and nervous system function. Found in whole grains, fruits, vegetables, and lean protein sources.

9.2 Caloric and nutrient intake: Understanding calorie needs and balancing nutrients

Finding the Right Balance:

- This is a guideline. Individual needs can vary based on factors like age, activity level, and dance style.
- Consulting a registered dietitian or sports nutritionist is highly recommended for a personalized plan.
- Track your intake: Utilize apps or food journals to monitor your calorie and nutrient intake. This helps identify areas for improvement.
- Fuel for performance: Eat a balanced meal 2-4 hours before practice to optimize energy levels.
- Refuel after workouts: Have a recovery snack within 30-60 minutes after dancing to replenish glycogen stores and aid muscle repair.

Remember:

Balance is key. By understanding your calorie needs and prioritizing the right mix of nutrients, you can fuel your body for peak performance as a dancer. Don't hesitate to seek professional guidance to create a personalized plan that takes your unique needs into account.

9.3 Nutrition and exercise: How your diet supports your dance training

Dancers push their bodies to the limit, demanding a diet that goes beyond just "healthy eating." Here's how the right nutrition supercharges your dance training:

Fueling Your Moves:

- **Energy Source:** Carbohydrates are the primary fuel for your muscles. Complex carbs like whole grains, fruits, and vegetables provide sustained energy to power through demanding routines. Simple carbs like sugary drinks or white bread offer a quick burst but can lead to crashes later.

- **Building Blocks**: Protein is crucial for muscle repair and growth. After intense training, your muscles undergo microscopic tears. Lean protein sources like chicken, fish, beans, and low-fat dairy help rebuild and strengthen your muscles, leading to improved performance.

- **Keeping You Going**: Healthy fats provide sustained energy, support hormone balance, and aid in vitamin absorption. Don't be afraid of healthy fats from nuts, seeds, avocados, and olive oil. These keep you fueled and feeling your best.

9.3 Nutrition and exercise: How your diet supports your dance training

Optimizing Performance:

- **Injury Prevention:** A balanced diet rich in calcium and Vitamin D strengthens bones, reducing the risk of stress fractures common in dance. Dairy products, leafy greens, fortified plant-based milk, and fatty fish are all excellent sources.

- **Enhanced Stamina:** Iron carries oxygen to your muscles, preventing fatigue. Foods like lean red meat, poultry, fish, beans, lentils, and dark leafy greens ensure your muscles get the oxygen they need to perform at their peak.

- **Sharpened Focus:** B vitamins support energy metabolism and nervous system function. Whole grains, fruits, vegetables, and lean protein sources are packed with B vitamins, keeping you sharp and focused during training.

Recovery and Repair:

- **Replenishing Stores:** After dancing, your glycogen stores (carbohydrate reserves) are depleted. Eating a recovery snack within 30-60 minutes with a combination of carbs and protein helps replenish these stores and kickstarts muscle repair.

9.3 Nutrition and exercise: How your diet supports your dance training

- **Hydration is Key:** Dancers lose a lot of fluids through sweat. Staying adequately hydrated is crucial for optimal performance and recovery. Aim to drink plenty of water throughout the day, even before feeling thirsty.

Remember:

- Listen to Your Body: Eat intuitively and adjust your portions based on your hunger cues and activity level.
- Individual Needs: This is a general guideline. A registered dietitian or sports nutritionist can create a personalized plan for your specific dance style and training intensity.

By prioritizing a balanced diet that aligns with your training demands, you can give your body the fuel it needs to excel. The right nutrition will not only improve your performance but also help you recover faster and prevent injuries, allowing you to dance your best.

9.4 Metabolism of dancers: The unique metabolic considerations for dancers

Dancers have a fascinating relationship with metabolism. Their bodies are finely tuned engines, burning a significant amount of calories during training and performances. However, there are unique metabolic considerations dancers need to be aware of to optimize their health and performance.

Burning Bright: The High-Performance Engine

- **Muscle Advantage:** Muscle tissue burns more calories at rest compared to fat tissue. Dancers, with their typically high muscle mass, have a naturally higher basal metabolic rate (BMR), meaning they burn more calories even when not actively dancing.

- **Energy Expenditure:** Dance training itself is a calorie-burning powerhouse. Depending on the style and intensity, dancers can burn anywhere from 400 to 1000 calories per hour. This high energy expenditure makes them efficient calorie burners.

9.4 Metabolism of dancers: The unique metabolic considerations for dancers

The Balancing Act: Challenges and Considerations

- **Undereating and the Metabolism Trap:** Despite burning a lot, some dancers may fall into the trap of restricting calories. This can backfire, causing the body to slow down its metabolism to conserve energy. The result? Fatigue, impaired performance, and increased risk of injury.

- **Nutrient Deficiencies:** Strict calorie restriction can also lead to deficiencies in essential nutrients like vitamins, minerals, and protein. These deficiencies can further hinder performance and recovery.

- **Stress and Hormones:** The pressure to maintain a certain physique or the demands of intense training can increase stress hormones like cortisol. Elevated cortisol can lead to muscle breakdown and hinder metabolism.

Optimizing Your Dance Metabolism

- **Fuel for the Fire:** Focus on a balanced diet that provides adequate calories, carbohydrates, protein, and healthy fats. Don't be afraid to eat enough to support your training!

- **Nutrient Timing:** Strategically timing your meals and snacks can optimize your metabolism. Aim for a balanced meal 2-4 hours before practice and a recovery snack with carbs and protein within 30-60 minutes after dancing.

- **Hydration Matters:** Dehydration can negatively impact metabolism. Stay adequately hydrated throughout the day to function at your best.

- **Prioritize Sleep:** Adequate sleep (7-8 hours) is crucial for recovery and helps regulate hormones that influence metabolism.

- **Listen to Your Body:** Don't ignore hunger cues. Eat intuitively and adjust portions based on your activity level.

Seeking Professional Guidance:

A registered dietitian or sports nutritionist can create a personalized plan that considers your dance style, training intensity, and individual needs. They can help you find the right balance of calories and nutrients to optimize your performance and maintain a healthy metabolism.

Remember:

Dancers have unique metabolic needs. By understanding these needs and prioritizing a balanced diet, adequate rest, and stress management, they can fuel their bodies for peak performance and maintain a healthy, well-functioning metabolism.

9.5 Controlling metabolism for dancers with diet and nutrition: Strategies for healthy weight management

Dancers are constantly striving for peak performance, and weight management plays a crucial role. However, crash diets and restrictive eating are counterproductive. Here's how to manage weight healthily through smart diet and nutrition choices:

Focus on Nutrient Density, Not Just Calories

- **Quality over Quantity:** Prioritize nutrient-dense whole foods like fruits, vegetables, whole grains, and lean protein sources. These foods provide essential vitamins, minerals, and fiber that keep you feeling full and support overall health.
- **Mindful Eating:** Pay attention to hunger cues and eat intuitively. Don't skip meals, as this can lead to overeating later. Savor your food and avoid distractions while eating.

9.5 Controlling metabolism for dancers with diet and nutrition: Strategies for healthy weight management

Fueling Your Body for Performance

- Carbohydrates: Your primary energy source. Complex carbs from whole grains offer sustained energy for rehearsals and performances. Aim for 55-60% of your daily calories from complex carbs.
- Protein: Essential for muscle repair and growth. Lean protein sources like chicken, fish, beans, and low-fat dairy help maintain muscle mass, which plays a vital role in metabolism. Aim for 15-20% of your daily calories from protein.
- Healthy Fats: Don't be afraid of healthy fats! Fats provide energy, support hormone balance, and aid in vitamin absorption. Include healthy fats from nuts, seeds, avocados, and olive oil in your diet. Aim for 20-30% of your daily calories from healthy fats.

Strategies for Healthy Weight Management:

- Portion Control: Use smaller plates and bowls to manage portion sizes.
- Snack Smart: Choose healthy snacks like fruits with nut butter, yogurt with berries, or vegetable sticks with hummus.
- Stay Hydrated: Water is essential for various bodily functions, including metabolism. Drink plenty of water throughout the day.
- Strength Training: Incorporate strength training exercises alongside your dance routine. Muscle burns more calories at rest, contributing to healthy weight management.

9.5 Controlling metabolism for dancers with diet and nutrition: Strategies for healthy weight management

Seeking Professional Help:

- **Registered Dietitian:** A consultation with a registered dietitian can help create a personalized plan considering your dance style, training intensity, and individual needs.
- **Body Composition Analysis:** Understanding your body composition (muscle mass vs. fat mass) can be more helpful than just weight on a scale. A professional can guide you on interpreting this data.

Remember:

The goal is not just weight loss, but healthy weight management. By focusing on a balanced diet, portion control, and adequate hydration, you can achieve healthy body composition while optimizing your performance. Don't be afraid to seek professional guidance to create a sustainable and healthy plan specifically tailored to your needs as a dancer.

www.ingramcontent.com/pod-product-compliance
Lightning Source LLC
Chambersburg PA
CBHW061248250726

48653CB00002B/568